DICTIONARY

OF

THE BACH FLOWER REMEDIES®

POSITIVE AND NEGATIVE ASPECTS

T. W. HYNE JONES

First published in Great Britain by

THE C. W. DANIEL COMPANY LTD.

1 Church Path, Saffron Walden, Essex, England

© Bach Flower Remedies Ltd.

ISBN 0 85207 145 0

First Edition 1976
Reprinted 1977
Reprinted 1978
Revised edition 1982
Reprinted 1983
Revised edition 1984
Reprinted 1985 (twice)
Reprinted 1986
Reprinted 1987 (twice)
Made and printed in Great Britain by
Hillman Printers (Frome) Ltd, Frome, Somerset

This simple Dictionary has been compiled to enable users and prescribers of the Bach Flower Remedies to make prompt comparative references and thus enhance their conclusions.

The Editor has found value in setting out both Negative and Positive manifestations alongside each other as the latter can often rank equally in importance, especially when the Remedies are combined. Some consideration given to the 'Positives invariably improves prescribing and results.

Material has been derived from various publications, practitioners' observations and from personal experience. The Editor is grateful for the many benefits from the Bach Remedies, for advice and encouragement given by the late Nora Weeks and other friends.

Tom Hyne Jones.

NOTES:

1) An asterisk * after the Remedy indicates Dr. Bach's twelve original Remedies.

2) The page number indicates the Remedy's alphabetical and numerical order.

3) Generally it can be taken that a person categorized by the 'Positive' aspect would have little need of the Remedy.

4) Some states of mind or condition can be aided by more than one remedy depending on the origin of the condition, e.g. sleeplessness might require Agrimony, White Chestnut or perhaps Vervain, hence in this book certain conditions being repeated under more than one heading. Please refer to each suggestion in turn in either the Handbook or Twelve Healers to determine the most suitable to the case in question.

5) Full information, explanatory literature, advice and treatment (if desired) can be obtained from: The Dr. Edward Bach Centre, Mount Vernon, Sotwell, Wallingford, Oxon OX10 0PZ, England. (SAE will be appreciated.)

AGRIMONY*

Keywords: MENTAL TORTURE BEHIND 'BRAVE FACE'

Negative

Carefreeness masks mental torture — a turbulent state of mind.

Seeks excitement the consequences of which can be dangerous and may bring harm.

Restless at night. Caused by churning thoughts. (See also White Chestnut.)

Dislikes being alone — may seek companionship in order to escape from and to forget worries.

Under stress, can resort to alcohol or drugs in order to dull mental torture.

Positive

Cheerful, carefree, a fine sense of humour, without pretence.

A good companion.

Can laugh at his own worries.

In illness, makes light of discomfort, even pain.

Distressed by quarrels and arguments. Peace loving. A peacemaker.

A genuine optimist.

ASPEN

Keywords: VAGUE FEARS OF UNKNOWN ORIGIN

Negative

Fears, by day or night, for *no known* reason. Apprehension. Terror on awakening – from a bad dream, although forgotten. Fear of going to sleep again. Terrible foreboding.

Some examples:

>   Fear of darkness.
>
>   Fear of death.
>
>   Fear of thoughts of disaster.
>
>   Fear when alone, or suddenly, when among friends – inexplicable.
>
>   Fear of fear. Afraid to tell her troubles to others.
>
>   Fears often accompanied by sweating and trembling.

Positive

Fearlessness, because the power of love stands behind and overcomes all things.

Once realised, we are beyond pain, suffering, care, worry, fear and become participants of true joy.

Such faith causes a desire for adventure, for experiences with disregard for difficulty or danger.

BEECH

Keyword: INTOLERANCE

Negative

Intolerance. Does not try to understand or make allowances for shortcomings of others.

Critical. Lacking in humility and sympathy.

Annoyed at small habits, mannerisms, idiosyncrasies and gestures of others.

Must have exactness, order and discipline everywhere.

A taskmaster. Complains about others.

Keeps to himself, lonely.

Positive

Strong convictions.

High ideals.

Although much appears to be wrong, there is ability to see good growing within.

Desire to be more tolerant, lenient and understanding towards others.

Dr. Bach's view of a perfect example of tolerance was Jesus Christ being crucified. He had no harsh thought and even pleaded for his malefactors.

CENTAURY*

Negative

Timid, easily imposed upon.

Little strength of will.

Doesn't argue or stand up for self – a 'door mat'. Cannot say 'no'.

Thoughts, actions often coloured by dictates and ideas of others and by conventions.

May be bound to family or parent. Servile instead of being a willing helper.

Positive

One who serves *wisely* and quietly.

One who knows when to give or when to withhold.

One who has strong individuality, is able to mix well and support his own opinions.

CERATO*

Negative

Doubts own ability.

Seeks advice from one and all, often influenced and misguided by advice of others which can cause dissatisfaction but needs their attention.

Lacks confidence in own judgement.

Distrusts own convictions. Changeable.

Foolish.

Talkative. Always asking questions.

Tends to sap vitality of others by seeking advice.

Has tendency to imitate.

Positive

Much wisdom, intuitive, holds definite opinions and will stick to a decision once arrived at.

Admires those who have a strong mind and can decide well and quickly.

CHERRY PLUM

Keywords: FEAR OF MIND GIVING WAY

Negative

Desperation.

Verge of nervous breakdown. Near hysteria – can shout for help.

Fear of suicide.

Fear that mind will give way to doing fearful things.

Fear of losing control and reason.

Fear of insanity.

Possibility of sudden murderous and violent impulses.

Positive

Calm, quiet courage.

Able to retain sanity despite mental and physical tortures, e.g. a prisoner of war.

CHESTNUT BUD

Keywords: FAILURE TO LEARN FROM PAST MISTAKES

Negative

Takes a long time to learn by experience – sometimes fails to do so.

Repeats making the same error.

Compulsive repetition of what has already been told.

Tries to forget the past but has no guide to help now or in the future. A pitiful situation until mistakes are recognised and thus avoided.

Positive

Keenly observant – of mistakes.

Gains knowledge and wisdom from experience.

Watches and learns from others.

Dr. Bach wrote: 'This Remedy is to help us to take full advantage of our daily experiences, and to see ourselves and our mistakes as others do.'

CHICORY*

Keywords: POSSESSIVE – SELFISH

Negative

Possessive love.

Easily feels hurt and offended and rejected.

Requires others to conform to their 'high sense of values' especially those near and dear. Interfering.

constant attention.

Talks of 'duty owed to him'.

When thwarted, becomes fretful, even tearful. Poisoned by such emotions.

Dislikes being alone.

Selfish, deceitful, strongwilled, talkative, irritable, enjoys arguments.

Positive

Selfless care and concern for others.

Always giving without any thought of return.

CLEMATIS*

Keywords: DREAMERS – LACK OF INTEREST IN PRESENT

Negative

Vacant look. Inattentiveness.

Pre-occupation. Indifference. Impractical type of person. Bemused, absent-minded. A dreamer.

Drowsiness. A heavy sleeper.

Enjoys dozing at any time – falls asleep easily. Listless.

Prefers to be alone. Avoids difficulties by withdrawing.

Positive

A lively interest in all things.

Sensitive to inspiration.

Idealistic – a writer, artist, actor, healer.

Master of his own thoughts.

Purposeful. Realistic. 'Down to earth.'

CRAB APPLE

Keywords: SELF-HATRED – SENSE OF UNCLEANLINESS

Negative

Feeling of despair, uncleanness, disgust. Has said or done something contrary to true nature.

Feels mentally and physically unclean. Ashamed of physical condition and appearance.

Despondent if treatment fails (see also Gentian). Has trivial thoughts – a 'bee in bonnet' – fussy – house proud.

Positive

The Cleansing Remedy for mind and body. Assistance against pollution and contamination. For internal and external use.

Ability to control thoughts and recognise difficulties and be acceptable again to oneself.

Can see things in correct perspective. Broadminded.

ELM

Negative

Sudden feeling of being overwhelmed by responsibilities and being inadequate for them.

Consequential despondency and exhaustion with ideas of being unequal to the job.

Even momentary doubt of abilities causes weakness and debility.

But all symptoms are only temporary.

Positive

Capable, efficient, intuitive.

Key positions in State or Industry – Physicians, Clergy, Teachers etc.

Leaders, decision-makers.

Positive awareness of responsibilities.

People of faith – confident self-assured.

Abilities usually directed towards the safety, welfare and betterment of others.

11

GENTIAN*

Keyword: DISCOURAGEMENT – DESPONDENCY

Negative

Negative outlook. Melancholy. Discouraged when things go wrong or when there are difficulties.

Despondent and depressed at setbacks from a KNOWN cause.

Refusal to believe that it is one's own lack of faith and understanding that prevents overcoming problems.

Failure to comprehend one's own negative mentality attracts these conditions of despondency and melancholia.

Remedy to help discouraged schoolchildren.

Positive

There's *no* failure when doing one's utmost.

No obstacle too great. No task too big.

Great conviction of accomplishments and of surmounting difficulties.

Not affected by setbacks.

A good convalescing tonic when indicated.

GORSE

Keywords: HOPELESSNESS – DESPAIR

Negative

Hopelessness. Despair, after being told 'nothing more can be done'.

Must continue to bear pain and suffering; may be convinced of inherited condition.

Almost useless to try different treatments.

Positive

Positive faith and hope.

Uninfluenced by present mental or physical condition or by other people's views.

Convinced that all difficulties will be overcome in the end.

Gorse is of value when given early in any chronic case.

Gives patient hope of recovery and that is the first step towards a cure.

HEATHER

Keywords: SELF-CENTREDNESS, SELF-CONCERN

Negative

Self-centredness. Self-concern.

'Obsessed' by ailments, problems and their trivia. Always wanting to tell others about them and about themselves. Sometimes weepy.

Comes close – speaks close into your face – 'buttonholers'.

Saps vitality of others, consequently is often avoided.

Dislikes being alone.

Makes mountains out of molehills.

A poor listener – has little interest in problems of others.

Positive

Restores vitality sapped by another.

A selfless, understanding person.

Because of having suffered, is willing to listen and help.

Can be absorbed in other's problems and is unsparing in efforts to help.

14

HOLLY

Keywords: HATRED, ENVY, JEALOUSY

Negative

Hatred, Envy, Jealousy, Suspicion, Aggressiveness, Greed.

Absence of love. Misunderstanding. Bad temper. Various forms of vexation. Anger towards fellow man.

Suffers much – often without a cause.

Positive

Protects from Hatred and from everything that is not of love.

Those of generous mind who are able to give without thought of recompense. Can rejoice in success of others. Willingness to share; not greedy nor possessive despite vexations and personal loss. Understanding, tolerant.

HONEYSUCKLE

Keywords: LIVES IN PAST

Negative

Nostalgia, Homesickness.

Lives in past. Has regrets.

In looking back, there is fear of what lies ahead; a 'state of Lot's wife', a 'torn-in-half' condition.

Can lose interest in present.

Slowing down of vital forces.

Positive

Overpowering past is now seen as an experience of essential value which can be laid to rest so that one can progress mentally and spiritually.

The Remedy for *memories* – of great help to widows, orphans, people who have failed in business etc., and especially to the older folk who have to live alone.

HORNBEAM

Keywords: 'MONDAY MORNING' FEELING

Negative

Weariness – mental fatigue.

Doubts strength to face or to *cope,* but usually accomplishes.

Convalescents doubt strength to recover.

Tiredness through self-preoccupation.

The Remedy for 'Monday morning' or 'Morning after'.

Positive

Certain of own ability and strength to face problems and what at first might appear to be insurmountable difficulties.

The Remedy that gives strength to those who feel weary in mind and body, and cannot cope with things of the moment.

IMPATIENS*

Keyword: IMPATIENCE

Negative

Irritable. Impatient. Nervous.

Everything done quickly.

A relief for mental tension through frustration.

Finishes sentence for the other person if slower.

Accident-prone through impetuosity.

Prefers to work alone.

Slow workers irritate.

Mental tension through frustration and other pressures.

Positive

Less hasty in action and thought. More relaxed, patient, tolerant and gentle towards shortcomings of others and 'upsetting conditions'.

LARCH

Keywords: LACK OF CONFIDENCE

Negative

No self-confidence. Useful before exams.

Convinced of failure, even to try.

Will never be a success.

Cannot do as well as others.

Feels inferior and possesses a false modesty (secretly knows ability is there).

'Admires' success of others without envy or jealousy simply because by standing down themselves the possibility of failure is averted.

Positive

Not fearful of failure *or* success.

Not frightened. Determined.

Capable.

Willing to 'plunge in' and take risks. Never discouraged by results.

Doesn't know meaning of the word 'can't'.

19

MIMULUS*

Keywords: FEAR OF KNOWN THINGS

Negative

Fear from *known* reasons.
Examples:
    Fear of illness and consequences.
    Fear of death.
    Fear of accidents – of pain.
    Fear of dark, of damp and cold.
    Fear of poverty.
    Fear of people – of animals.
    Fear of speaking in public.
    Fear of losing friends.

Secret fears, is tongue-tied, has stage-fright.

Blushes easily – may suffer from stammering. Shyness. Timidity.

Possesses love and understanding which can overcome things disliked and not understood.

Positive

Quiet courage to face trials and difficulties with equanimity and humour.

Emotions completely under control – ability to enjoy life once more without irrational fears.

MUSTARD

Keywords: DEEP GLOOM WITH NO ORIGIN (BLACK DEPRESSION)

Negative

Descending gloom. **Hopeless, despairing depression and melancholia which comes suddenly and lifts just as suddenly *without apparent reason*.**

The *gloom,* as if overshadowed by a cold, dark cloud, can be very severe depriving the sufferer of normal cheerfulness and thoughts, for they are all turned upon himself.

Positive

Inner serenity, stability, joy and peace that nothing can shake or destroy.

OAK

Negative

Overworks and hides tiredness. Plodders. Despondency leading to despair. Obstinate, relentless effort, although it may have become useless; could eventually result in a nervous breakdown.

Positive

Has courage and is stable under all conditions.

Likes helping others. Reliable.

Strong, patient, full of common sense, can stand great strain.

The Oak people are brave, and fight adversity, difficulties and illness without loss of hope. They persevere and are ceaseless in their effort to find a cure when unwell.
(Although this is a positive description – it is when the inner strength begins to wane and collapse thus creating tiredness and signs of losing the battle that OAK is needed.)

OLIVE

Keywords: COMPLETE EXHAUSTION

Negative

Suffered long under adverse conditions, or vitality has been sapped from a long illness.

Mind wearied and exhausted.

No reserve strength. Everything an effort. Tires easily. Lack of zest. Total fatigue of mind and body.

Little time for relaxation and enjoyment.

Cannot enjoy work or things that used to give pleasure and interest.

Positive

Remedy for convalescence.

Remedy of applied faith, i.e. non-reliance on personal effort to overcome.

Remedy to restore peace of mind, vitality, strength and interest.

Claim of strength and vitality to sustain and guide others in need.

Ability to maintain peace, harmony and interest 'even though one may be forced to remain inactive'.

PINE

Keywords: SELF REPROACH – GUILT

Negative

Self-reproach. Blames self for mistakes of others and for everything that goes wrong.

Has guilt-complex which takes away all joy.

Is over-conscientious but never content with achievements and often overworks.

Positive

Takes responsibility with a fair and balanced attitude.

Great perseverance, humility, and sound judgement.

Note: *Not to be confused with self disgust* (*see Crab Apple*).

RED CHESTNUT

Keywords: ANXIETY FOR OTHERS

Negative

Over concern and *fear for others* – of calamity befalling them – the worst.

Fear that a minor complaint in another person will become a serious one.

Such fearful, negative thoughts harm us and those around us.

Positive

Ability to send out thoughts of safety, health or courage to those who need them.

Ability to remain calm, mentally and physically, in any emergency.

ROCK ROSE*

Keyword: TERROR

Negative

The Remedy for rescuing from Terror – Panic.

From an accident or near escape.

From the spectacle of an accident.

Whenever there's terror in the atmosphere – both patient and those around are affected.

A child's terror from a nightmare (a few drops in a little water sipped frequently will quickly calm).

Positive

Great courage – is willing to risk life for others.

Self is forgotten. Strength of will and character.

ROCK WATER

Keywords: SELF REPRESSION AND DENIAL

Negative

Over-concentration on self.

A *taught tightened-up* person.

The Remedy for those with strong opinions and who allow their minds to be ruled by prized theories. *Rigidity* of outlook, often physical as well.

Hard taskmasters on themselves.

Self-denial – Self-domination, even Self-martyrdom.

They do not usually interfere in the lives of others because they are far too concerned with their own perfection and setting an example for all to behold.

Positive

Has high ideals – a flexible mind and one who is willing to forsake an original theory if a greater truth is revealed.

Has sufficient conviction not to be easily influenced by others.

Such joy and peace experienced, that others are encouraged to follow.

Some drops added to bath will help.

SCLERANTHUS*

Keywords: UNCERTAINTY – INDECISION

Negative

Indecision. Grasshopper mind. *Swayed between two possibilities.* Uncertainty.

Varying moods, light and shade.

Experiences extremes of: –
   Joy and Sadness
   Energy and Apathy
   Optimism and Pessimism
   Laughing and Crying

Can be unreliable – uncertain due to constantly changing outlook.

Wastes time and loses opportunities.

Lack of poise and balance.

Subject to car, air or seasickness.

Positive

Calmness. Determination.

Makes quick decisions.

Takes prompt action.

Keeps poise and balance under all occasions.

STAR OF BETHLEHEM

Keyword: SHOCK

Negative

SHOCK in any form —

An accident — sudden sad news.

A bad fright — a grievous disappointment.

Many unsuspected, delayed-action effects from shock.

Positive

Neutralises shock and the effect of shock whether immediate or delayed.

'The comforter and soother of pains and sorrows.'

SWEET CHESTNUT

Keywords: EXTREME ANGUISH

Negative

Terrible, appalling mental despair. Extreme mental torture. Anguish of bereavement.

Reached limit of endurance.

Almost destroyed. Exhaustion and loneliness is total.

Future is complete darkness. No hope – no peace.

Positive

Strong character.

Full control of emotions.

Likely to keep troubles to self.

Those who, despite unbearable anguish, can call on the Father for help and still put their trust in Him.

The cry for help is heard and miracles happen!

VERVAIN*

Keywords: TENSENESS – HYPERANXIETY

Negative

Extremes of mental energy – over-effort, stress.

Will forces actions beyond physical strength.

Tenseness causes inability to relax and subsequent sleeplessness.

'Runs a thing to death'. Highly strung – fanatical. Perfectionist. Sensitive to injustices.

Mind always ahead, inclined to tackle too many jobs at the same time.

Positive

One who teaches that great accomplishments are by Being rather than by Doing.

Great courage. Faces danger willingly to defend a cause.

Calm, wise and tolerant with ability to relax. Always ready to listen.

Holds strong opinions which rarely change *but is ready to do so if necessary*.

VINE

Keywords: DOMINEERING – INFLEXIBLE

Negative

Tendency to use great gifts to gain power and to dominate. Rides roughshod over others' opinions. Demands and expects absolute obedience. Aggressive pride.

Craves power – greedy for authority. Ruthless in methods. Knows better than anyone. Forces will upon one and all. Can be tyrannical and dictatorial. Enjoys power over others – is hard, cruel and without compassion.

A parent dominating the home with iron discipline.

Positive

A wise, loving, understanding ruler, leader or teacher. Very capable, confident and ambitious.

Uses his great qualities to guide without the need to dominate.

Helps others to know themselves and to find a path in life.

A leader who inspires others by his unshakable confidence and certainty.

WALNUT

Keywords: PROTECTION FROM CHANGE AND OUTSIDE INFLUENCES

Negative

Oversensitive to certain ideas, atmosphere and influences.

May be affected by a dominating personality, a forceful circumstance, a link with the past, a family tie or a binding habit, any of which situations can hinder and frustrate plans or even a course of life.

Positive

Ideals and ambitions – such as those of pioneers, inventors or explorers – with a constancy and determination to carry them out despite adverse circumstances, opinions and ridicule.

Walnut gives protection against the adverse effects of over-sensitivity to certain ideas, atmosphere and influences.
It is the Remedy for the transition stages in life – teething, puberty, menopause and is definitely the link-breaking, spell-breaking and bond-freeing remedy.
Walnut is of much value when making big decisions such as changing religion, occupation or when moving home.
When taking 'great steps forward', breaking away from old conventions, restrictions etc., and when starting a new Way, often with attendant sufferings of severance from valued associations.

33

WATER VIOLET*

Keywords: PROUD, ALOOF

Negative

Because of knowledge and capability, they sometimes appear to be proud, aloof, disdainful and condescending.

Such mental rigidity can create physical stiffness and tension.

Positive

They like to be alone and are independent, self-reliant.

Quiet, gentle, tranquil, sympathetic and wise people who have poise and dignity and put their capabilities to the service of others.

Bears grief and sorrows in silence.

In a normal state is willing to offer advice without becoming personally involved in the affairs of others.

WHITE CHESTNUT

Keywords: UNWANTED THOUGHTS, MENTAL ARGUMENTS

Negative

A worrying or distressing occurrence preys on the mind. Mental arguments.

Helpless to prevent thoughts going round and round in the mind like a hamster on a wheel.

Persistent, unwanted thoughts are like a gramophone record when the stylus has jumped the groove and invariably cause a troubled mind and sleeplessness.

This sufferer is pre-occupied, lacks concentration and often does not answer when spoken to, which state of mind could lead to accidents.

Positive

A quiet, calm mind – at peace with himself and others which enables him to control his thoughts, to put them to constructive use and to solve his problems.

WILD OAT

Keywords: UNCERTAINTY RE CORRECT PATH IN LIFE

Negative

Undecided as to what to do. Uncertainty (also see Scleranthus). Things not clear, causing despondency and dissatisfaction.

Talented and ambitious – tries many things but none brings happiness – becomes frustrated and depressed. Can feel bored.

Positive

Definite character, talents and ambitions.

Lives a life filled with usefulness and happiness.

Of assistance in selecting a career

WILD ROSE

Keywords: RESIGNATION, APATHY

Negative

Resigned to illness, monotony, uncongenial work. Too apathetic to get well, to change occupation or to enjoy simple pleasures, despite to do so lies in her hands. Drifter.

Resignation – surrender. 'I must learn to live with it'. 'It is in the family so I must expect to suffer'. Believes a condition is incurable.

Fails to realise she has actually created these conditions, nourishes and maintains them.

Always weary, lacking in vitality and makes a dull companion. May have monotonous expressionless voice.

Positive

Lively interest in all happenings.

Ambitious. Purposeful.

Interest and vitality produces happiness, the enrichment and enjoyment of friends and good health.

WILLOW

Keyword: RESENTMENT

Negative

Resentment – bitterness – self-pity – blames everyone but himself. 'I have not deserved this misfortune; why should it happen to me while others get off scot-free?'

Begrudges good-fortune, health, happiness or success of fellow men.

Irritable, sulky, a 'wet blanket' who enjoys spreading gloom and despair. A grumbler.

No interest in the affairs of others except to decry and to speak with unkindness.

Takes without giving – accepts help as a 'right' – ungrateful – alienating.

In sickness, a difficult patient; nothing pleases or satisfies.

Reluctant to admit improvement.

Positive

Optimism and faith.

One who recognises responsibilities and the power to attract good or bad according to the nature of his thoughts.

Most of us suffer more or less the negative mind of Willow at times, so this Remedy will neutralise and help us to regain a sense of humour and to see things in their true perspective.

THE RESCUE REMEDY®

For FIRST-AID use, EMERGENCIES AND ASSOCIATED STRESS

This is a composite of five Flower Remedies – *IMPATIENS, STAR OF BETHLEHEM, CHERRY PLUM, ROCK ROSE, and CLEMATIS* – discovered and used with great effect by the late Dr. Edward Bach.

If you have received a shock of any kind, some sudden bad news, if there has been a family upset or you are in sorrow such as before and at a funeral; if you are fearful or confused, even in terror or in a panic, Rescue Remedy will come to your aid by helping you to face up to these problems of stress.

When you are awaiting some important news, about to take exams, attend a difficult meeting or have an interview; if you are going on stage, speaking in public, about to take your driving test or going to the dentist or into hospital, Rescue Remedy will always help to relieve your apprehension; likewise, whenever you feel 'up-tight', tensed up or unduly bothered, it is a good natural healer and can usually restore your balance and confidence.

On occasions when your mind is over-active or not at peace take a dose or two in the evening and before going to sleep but do not expect Rescue Remedy to counteract automatically the disturbing effects of TV horror films and other exciting items seen and heard late at night – you must switch off in time!

In all these problems try to overcome them positively and use Rescue Remedy to assist your effort.

Many have proved that having Rescue available for immediate use to nullify the sufferer's shock and fear is of the utmost importance in helping the natural healing process of one's being to proceed without hindrance.

Rescue Remedy provides an effective treatment for stress particularly resulting from emergencies. If, for example, there has been a bad accident at home, out of doors or on the road, those involved may be experiencing one or more of these emotions: shock, fear, terror or panic, severe mental tension, a feeling of desperation or a numbed, bemused state of mind. In the circumstances a doctor should have been called immediately and while the giving of Rescue Remedy does not, nor is intended to take the place of medical attention, it possesses life-saving potentialities so that until the doctor's arrival it can relieve the sufferers' fear and help to restore calmness.

Treatment for Accidents:

Dosage for Rescue Remedy Stock (when used as a separate Remedy)

For immediate or emergency use, 4 drops in a small glass of water (can be taken in other liquids, e.g. fruit juice, various beverages) to be sipped frequently — replenish glass to continue treatment if necessary. If the sufferer is unable to swallow, or in a comatose state, then the lips, behind the ears and the wrists should be moistened with the Remedy.

It is always worthwhile to carry a small bottle with you in case of unexpected need.

EXTERNAL APPLICATION

'Rescue Remedy' cream can be applied to lacerations, bites, stings, burns, sprains, massage and many other needs.

The 'Rescue Remedy' liquid can be diluted and used externally as a lotion. A couple of undiluted drops direct from the bottle will also help above conditions, except of course where the skin is severely broken.

PLEASE NOTE:

Rescue is a natural remedy, it is entirely safe, it has no side effects nor is it habit-forming and it will not intefere with any other medical treatment.

Remember Rescue Remedy for your **pets, domestic animals** and any other living creatures; if they have suffered fright or injury 4 drops on food or in their drinking water can benefit them immensely. Repeat if necessary.

Similarly in the **garden** and **greenhouse.** If a tree or shrub has been transplanted it has received some shock; treatment for a day or two will reduce the effect and commence rejuvenation. Put 10 drops from the bottle into the watering-can and pour around the roots (if the ground is dry give a good watering beforehand). Use a fine spray for foliage. For pricked-out seedlings and potted-on plants put 4 drops in a Bio Mister hand sprayer and apply to compost and foliage.

Stock concentrates of all remedies, books, charts, illustrations and general information, including full dosage instructions and list of appointed foreign distributors available from:

Bach Flower Remedies Ltd,
The Dr. Edward Bach Centre,
Mount Vernon, Sotwell,
WALLINGFORD.
Oxon. OX10 0PZ.
Tel: Wallingford 39489 (line open
9.30 a.m.—3 p.m. Mon—Fri inclusive)

Other books about The Bach Flower Remedies

Introduction to the Benefits of the Bach Flower Remedies
Jane Evans

'There is a system of medicine discovered some thirty years ago, whereby disease can be prevented before its physical symptoms are made manifest, the use of which involves very little cost; perhaps that is why it is so little known . . .'

The Medical Discoveries of Edward Bach
Nora Weeks

The life and work of a great physician who combined compassion for all who suffered, with a deep love for Nature.

The Twelve Healers
Edward Bach

The simple method of healing through the personality by means of wild flowers for the lay healer and the home.

The Bach Remedies Repertory
F. J. Wheeler

This supplementary guide will assist those seeking to develop their own ability to choose and administer the right remedy.

Heal Thyself
Edward Bach

An explanation of the real cause and cure of disease. Dr. Bach shows the vital principles which will guide medicine in the near future, and are already guiding some of the more advanced members of the profession today

The Illustrated Handbook of the Bach Flower Remedies
Philip Chancellor

Practical information on prescribing with case histories. It now contains colour illustrations of all the Remedies from the water-colours of Marjorie Pemberton Pigott.

A Guide to the Bach Flower Remedies
Julian Barnard

The latest addition to the Bach Flower books and a practical comprehensive and concise guide for the layman. The contents include: How the Remedies Work, When We take the Remedy, Diagnosis and Prescribing, Combination Remedies, Dowsing, Learning to Diagnose and Making the Medicine.